The New Mama's

AFFIRMING COLORING BOOK

WRITTEN BY
LEAH HAIRSTON, MSSW

ILLUSTRATED BY
AKISTA HORTON

The New Mama's Affirming Coloring Book
Written by Leah Hairston, MSSW Illustrated by Akista Horton
Publisher: Soulcial Healing, LLC
Publication Date: May 5, 2023
ISBN: 979-8-218-20639-0
Cover Design: Leah Hairston, MSSW

Soulcial Healing, LLC
822 Guilford Avenue #740
Baltimore, MD 21202

This book is dedicated to all the mamas I've loved, those who have loved me, and all the Black mamas who will pick up this compilation of loving affirmations. You are seen and celebrated in all seasons of your journey. I hope you see yourself represented in this work.

I'd like to say a special thank you to my parents, Rod and Sheri Hairston, as well as my grandma, Betty Hairston-Boyd. Thank you for pouring your love and wisdom into me. My roots run deep because of you.

Also, thank you to Joy Gilmer-Marseille for making me a godmama. Thank you for your love, encouragement, and insights as I crafted this artistry. Tis blessed to have you as her mama. I'm honored to do life with y'all.

To my team, thank you for helping to bring this vision to life.

I USE MY INSTINCTS TO ASSIGN THE ROLES OF MY BIRTH TEAM.

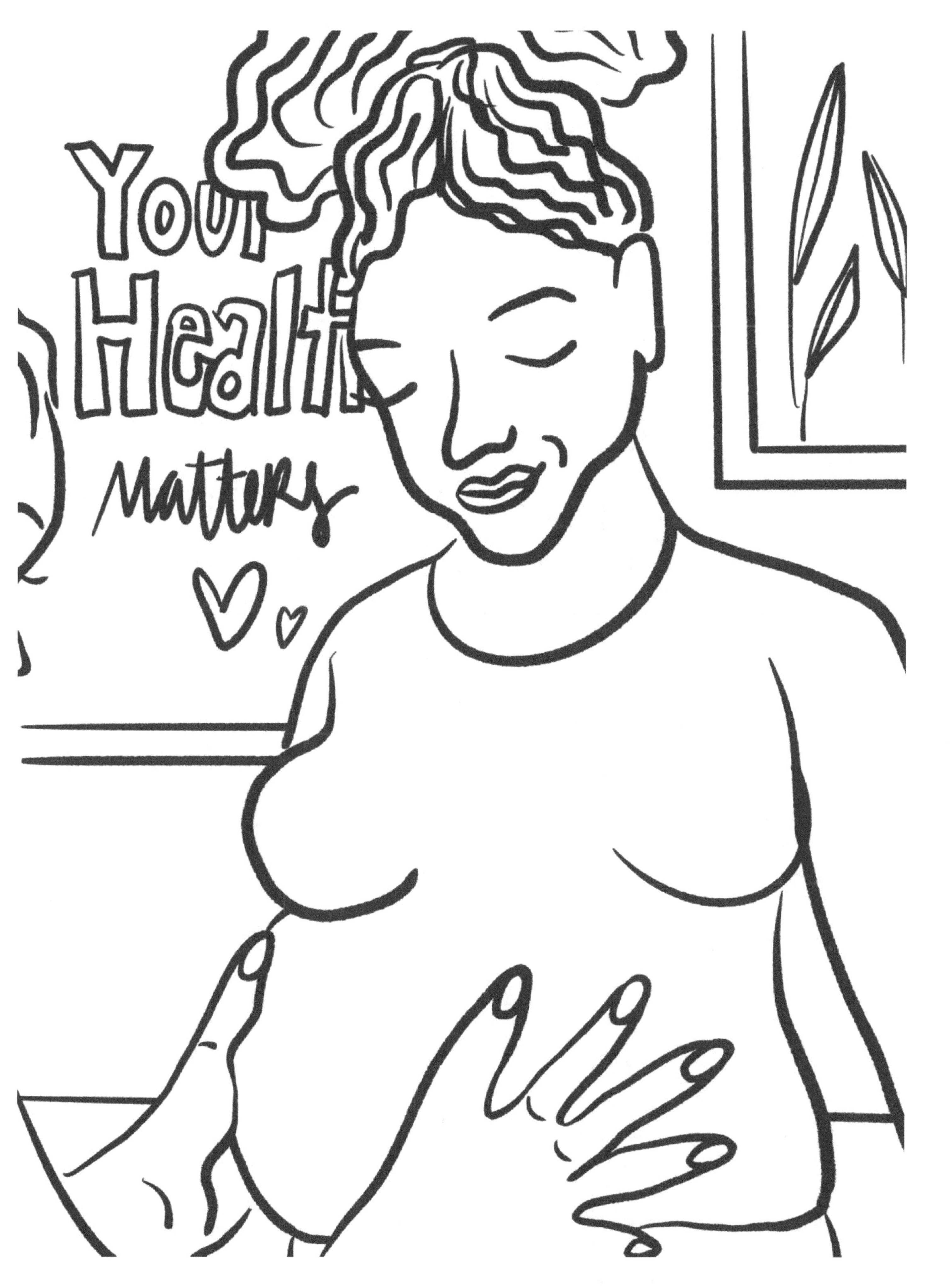

Your
Health
Matters

I

BREATHE

DEEPLY.

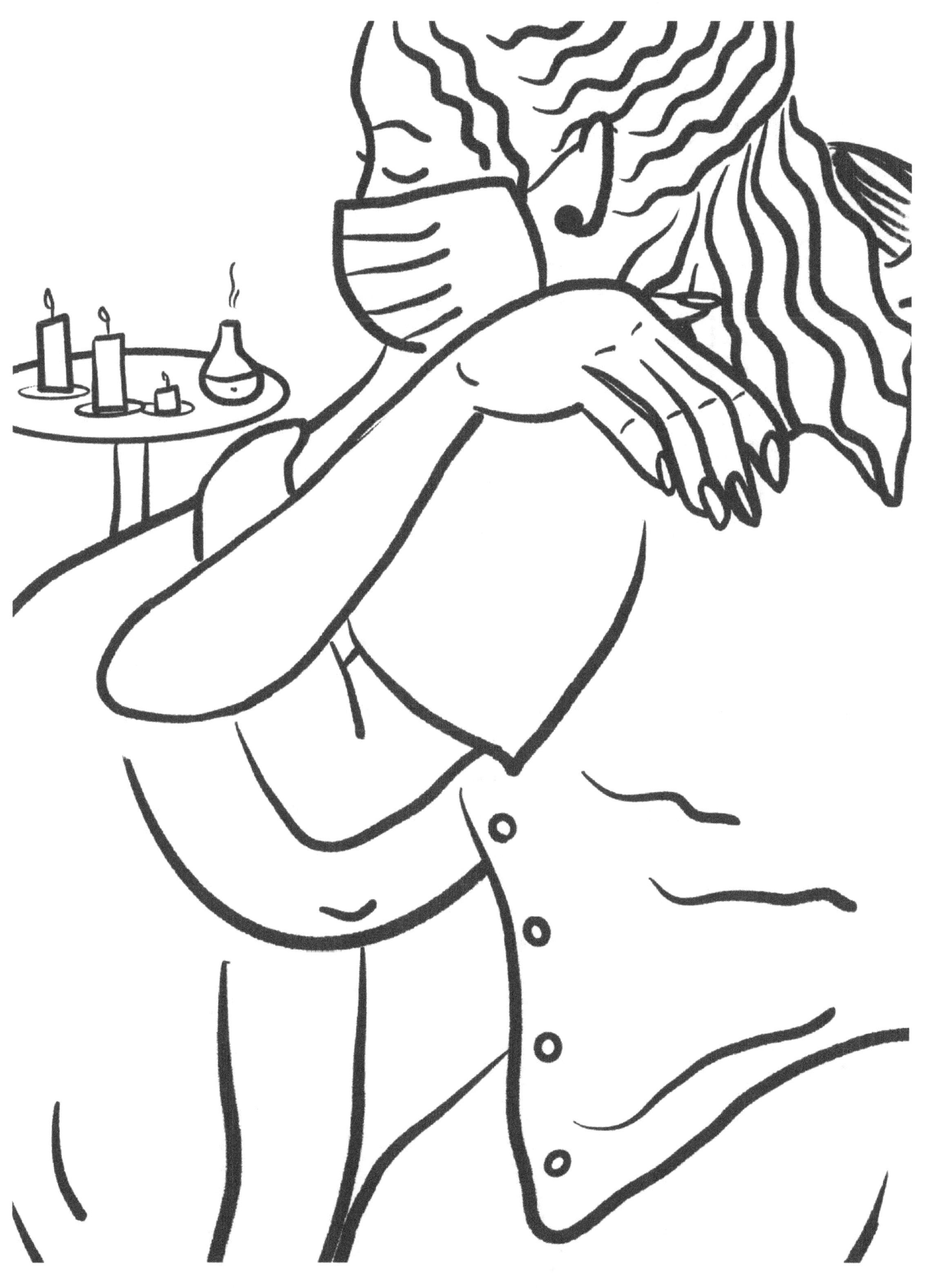

I TRUST MY INSTINCTS.

MY TEAM HONORS MY CHOICES.

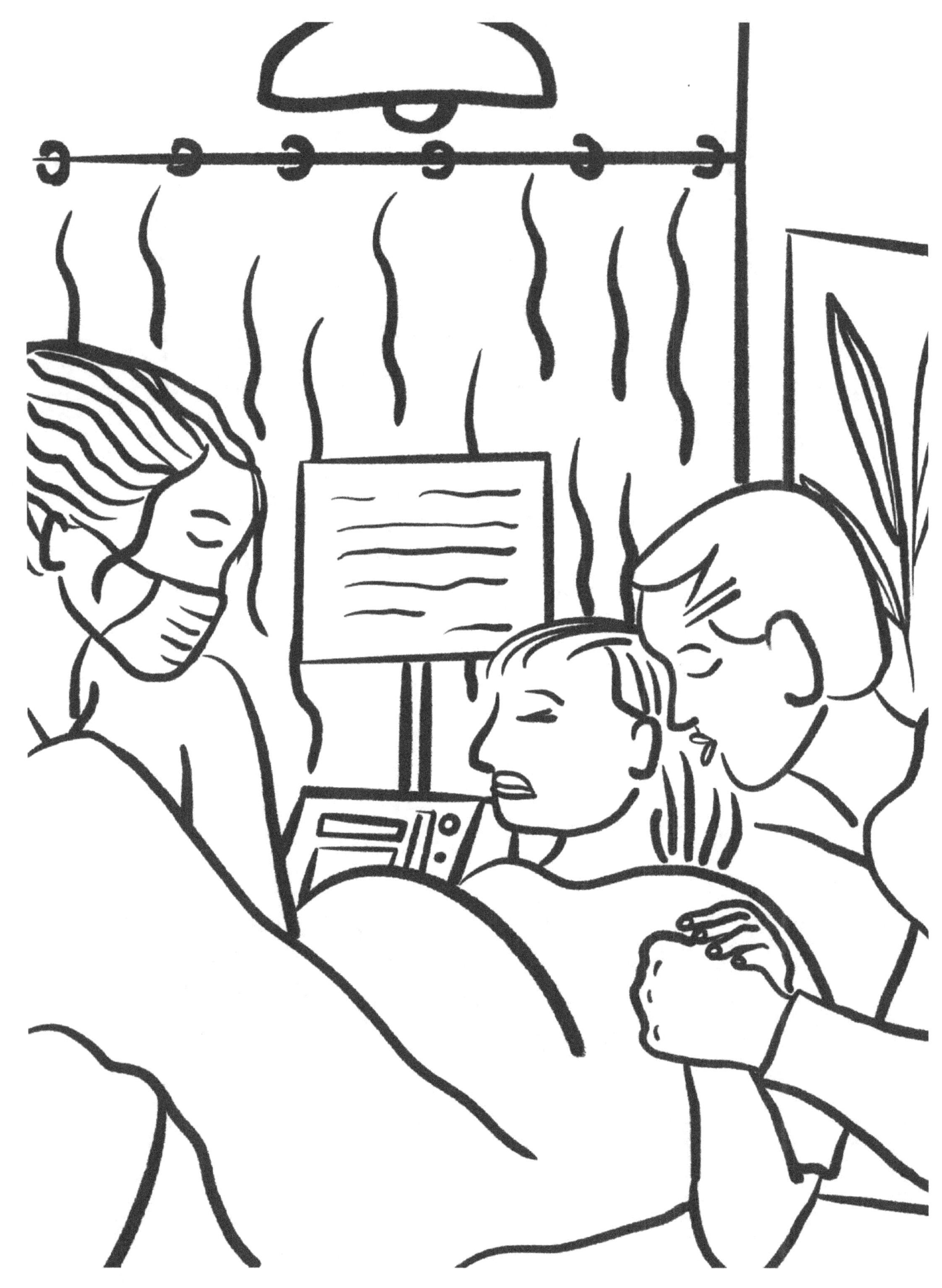

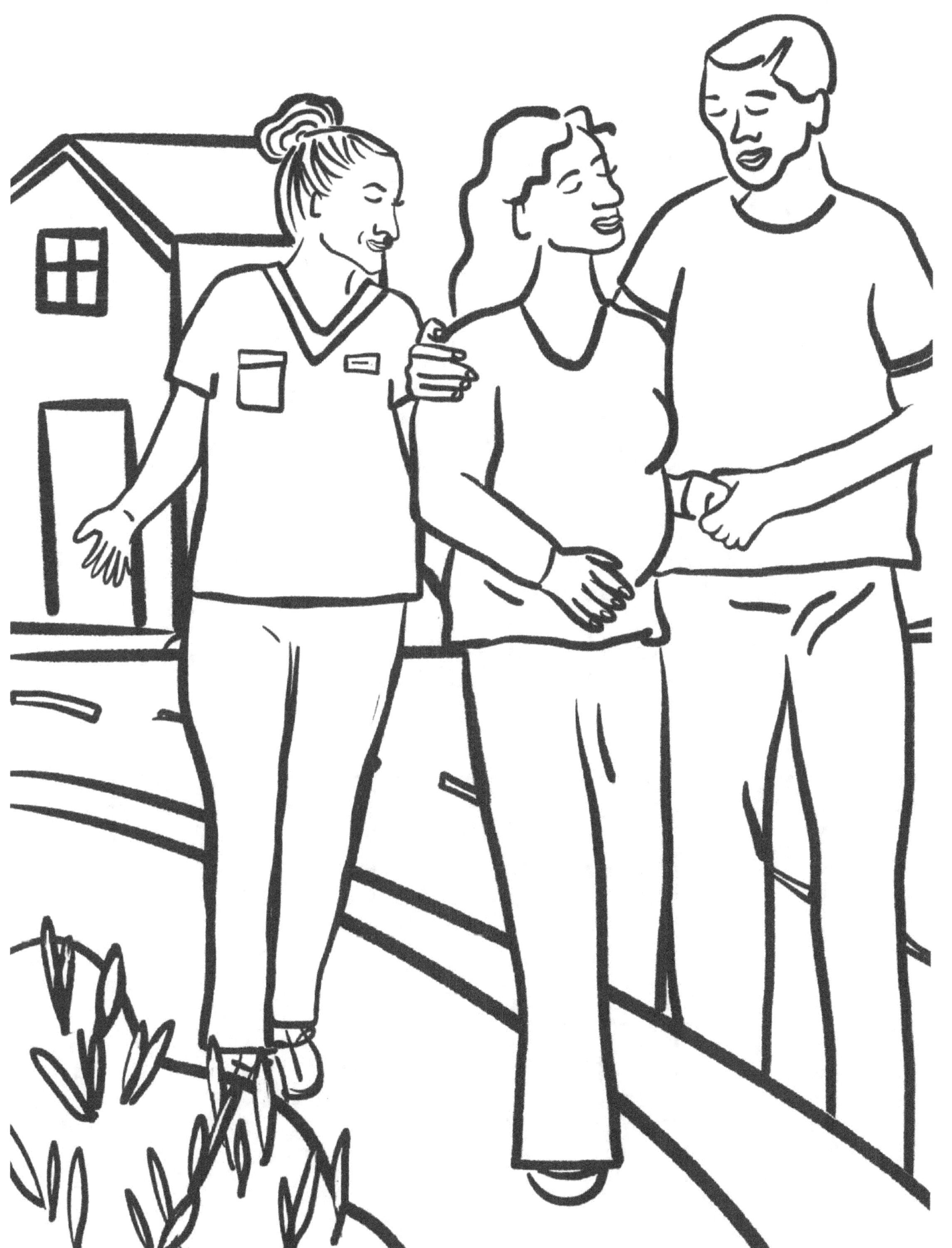

I USE MY VOICE TO CURATE MY BIRTH TEAM.

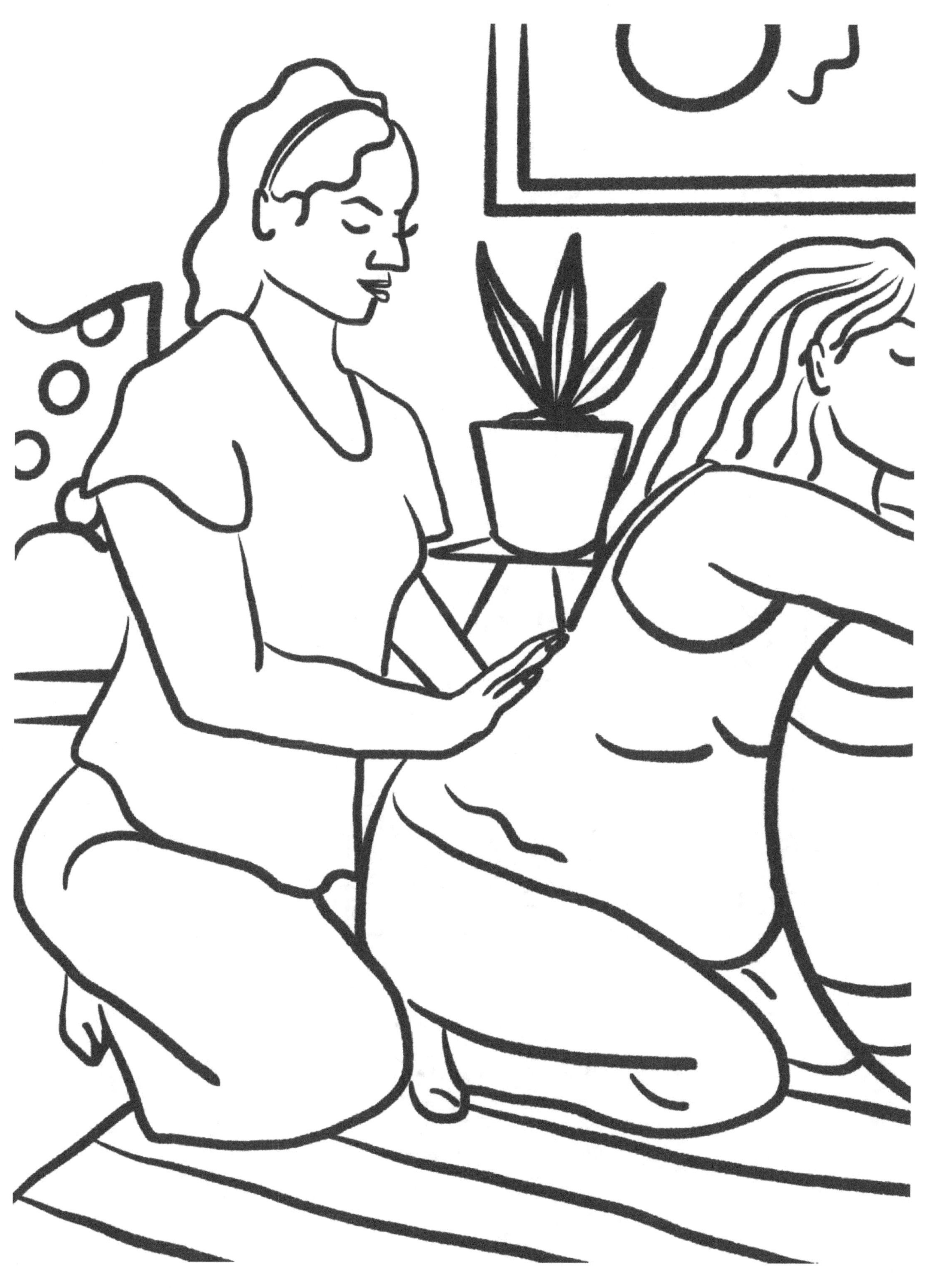

EACH WAVE BRINGS MY BABY CLOSER TO ME.

I CAN CREATE AN EMPOWERED BIRTH EXPERIENCE.

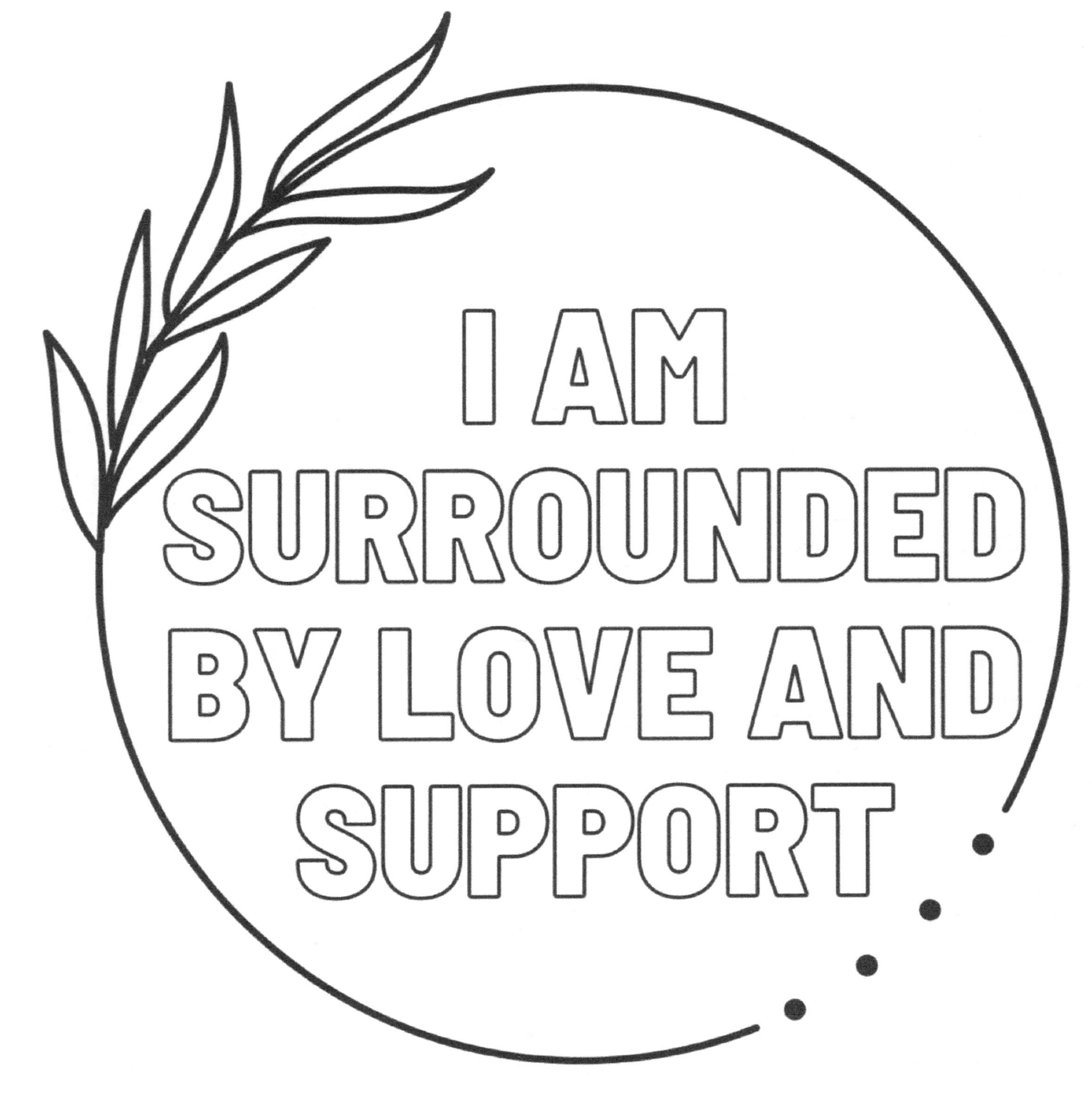

I AM
SURROUNDED
BY LOVE AND
SUPPORT

BIRTH IS A PROCESS I CHOOSE TO EMBRACE.

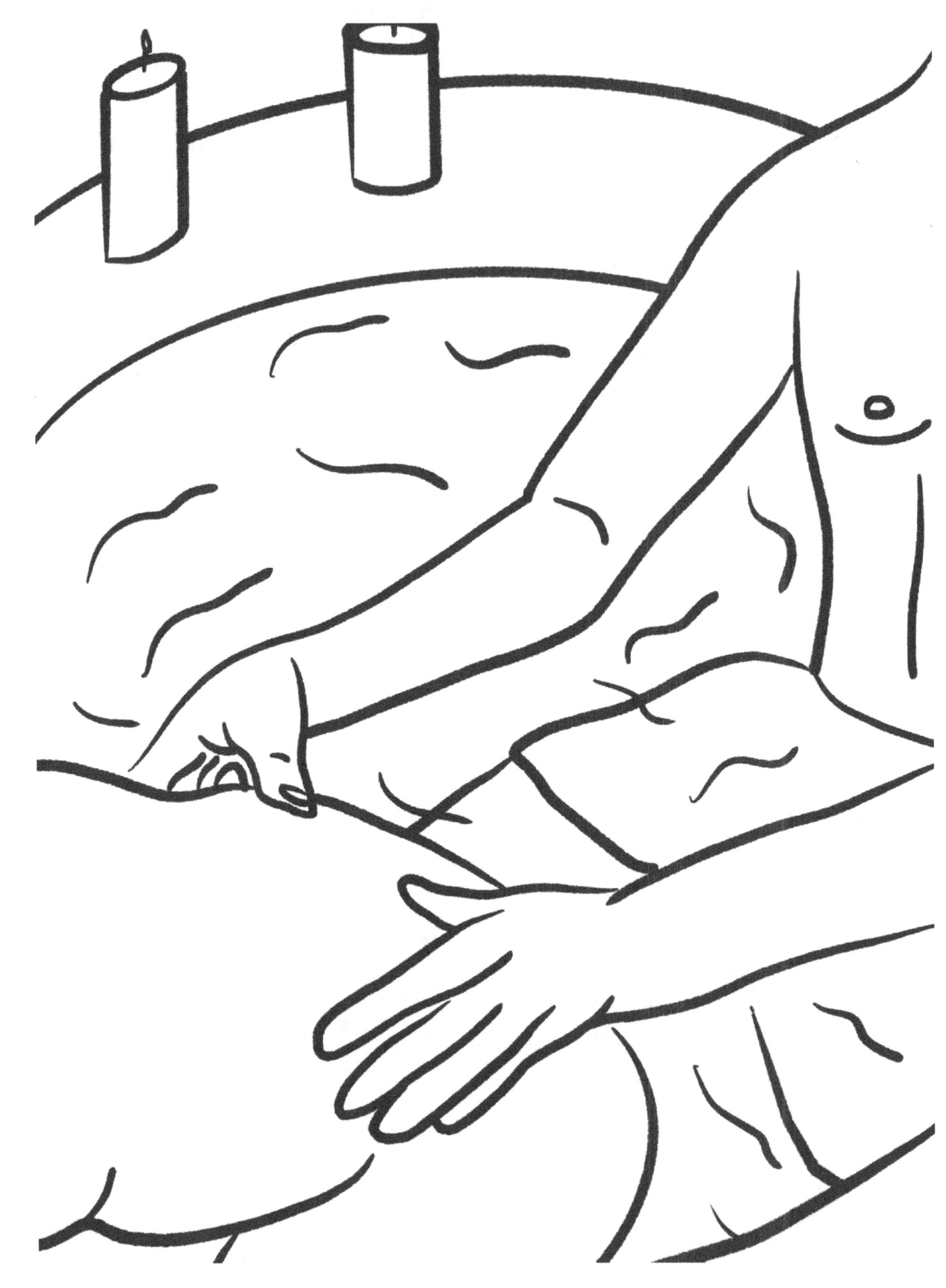

I EMBRACE THE JOURNEY OF LEARNING MY BABY.

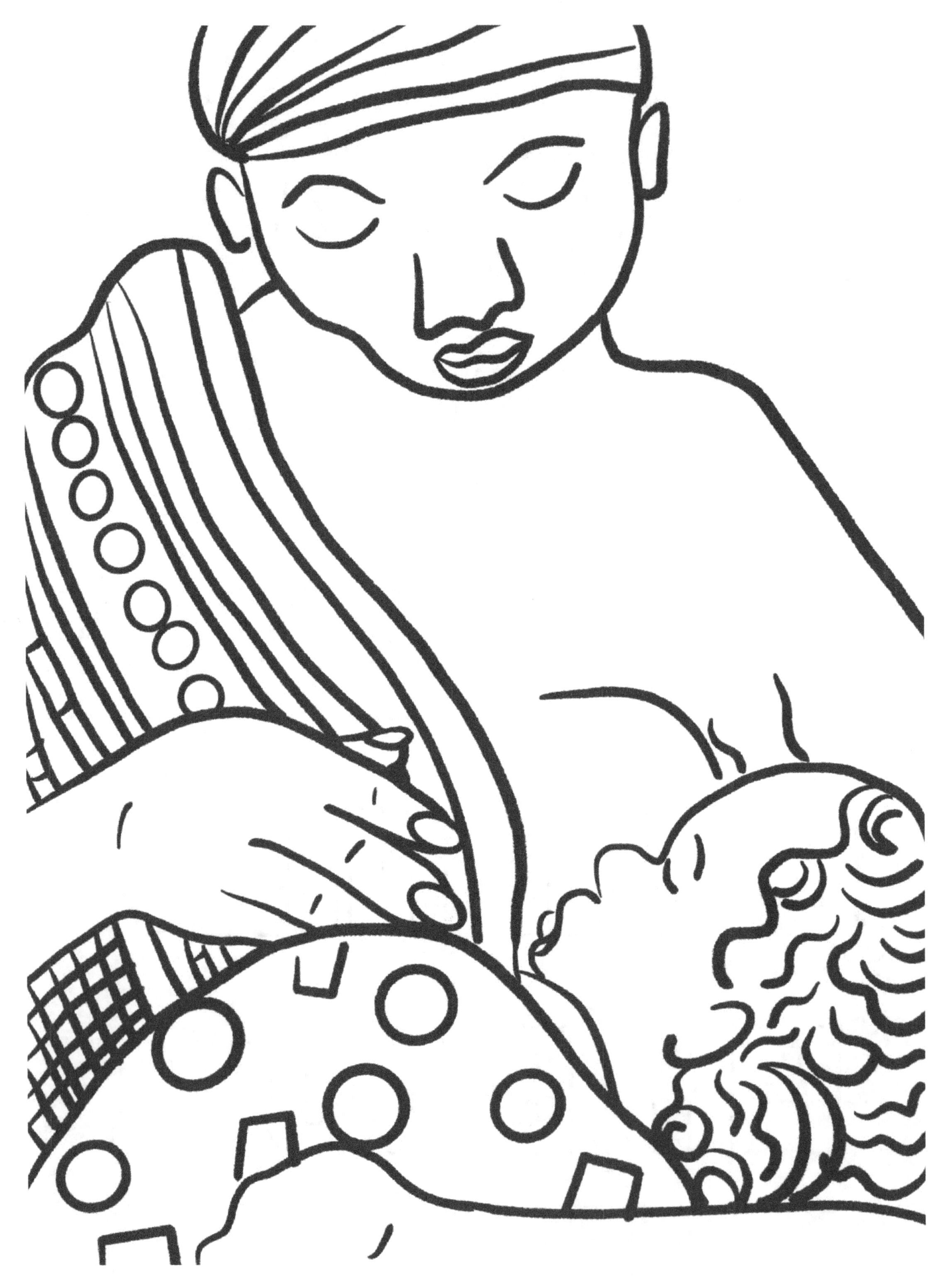

I CHOOSE TO NOURISH MY BODY.

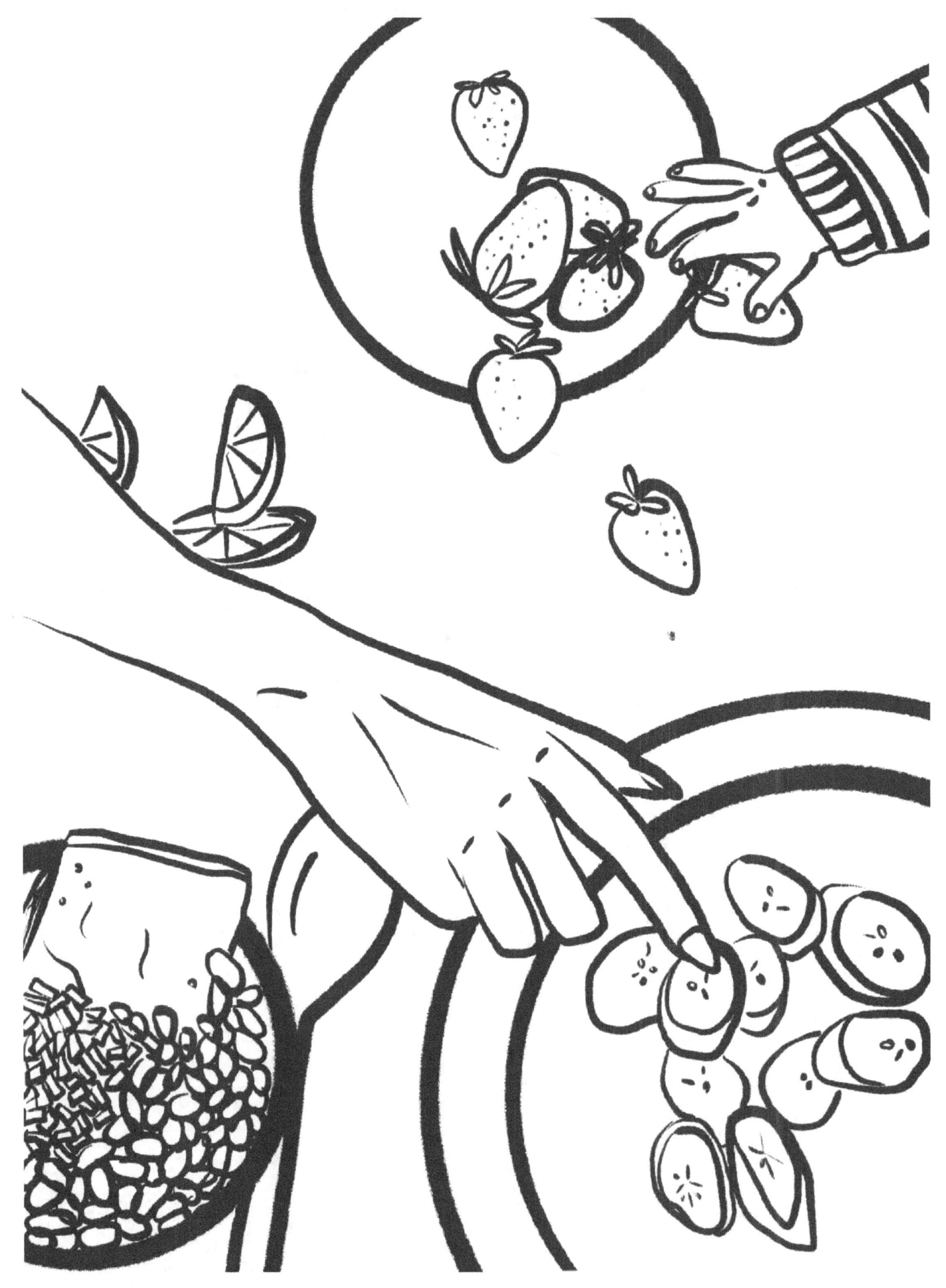

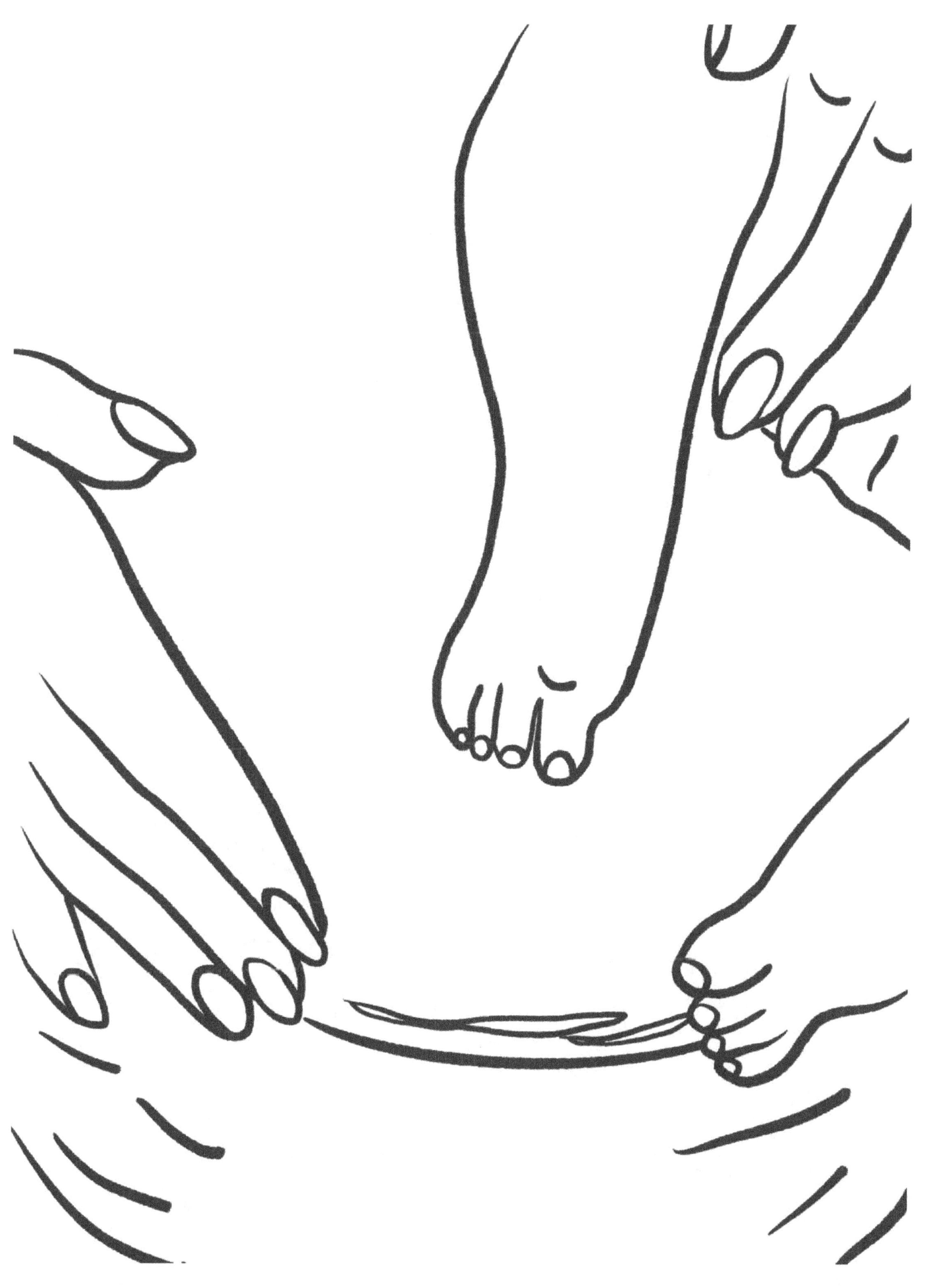

MY BIRTH STORY MATTERS. EVEN IF IT WAS NOT WHAT I PLANNED.

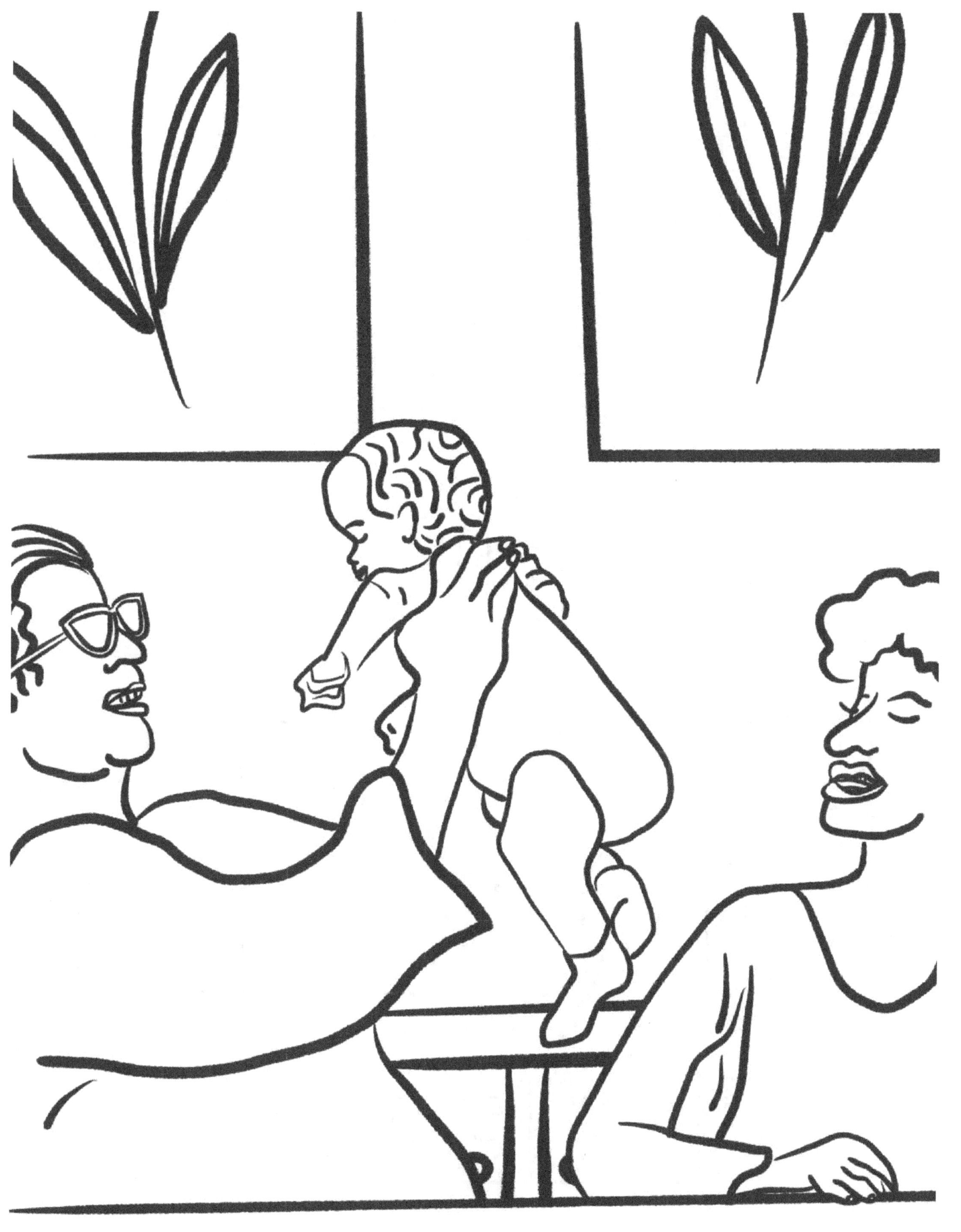

I USE MY VOICE SO I CAN LET OTHERS KNOW WHAT I NEED.

I EMBRACE THIS JOURNEY.

I SURRENDER TO THE NEWNESS.

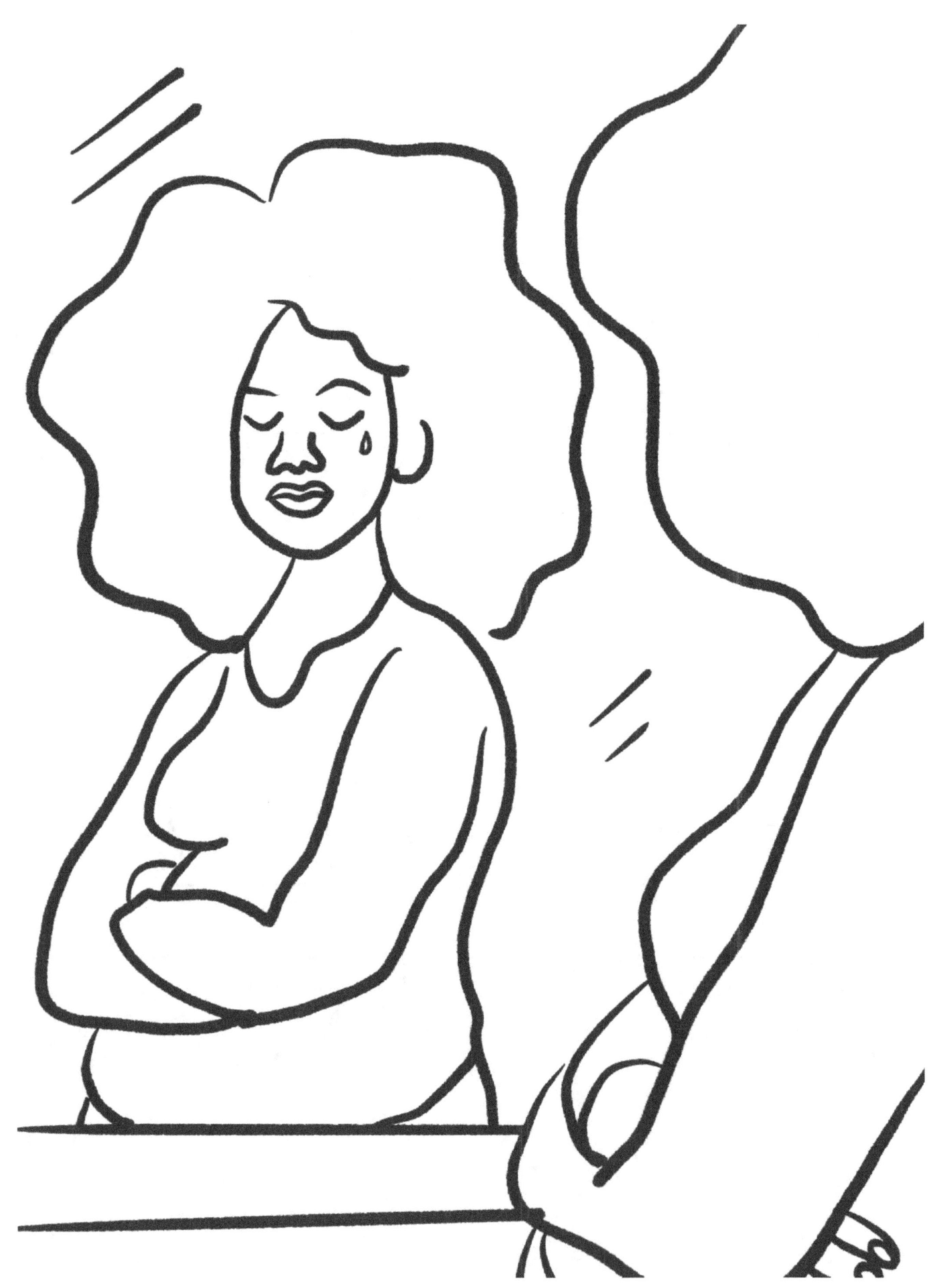

MY BABY
TRUSTS ME.
I WILL
TRUST ME TOO.

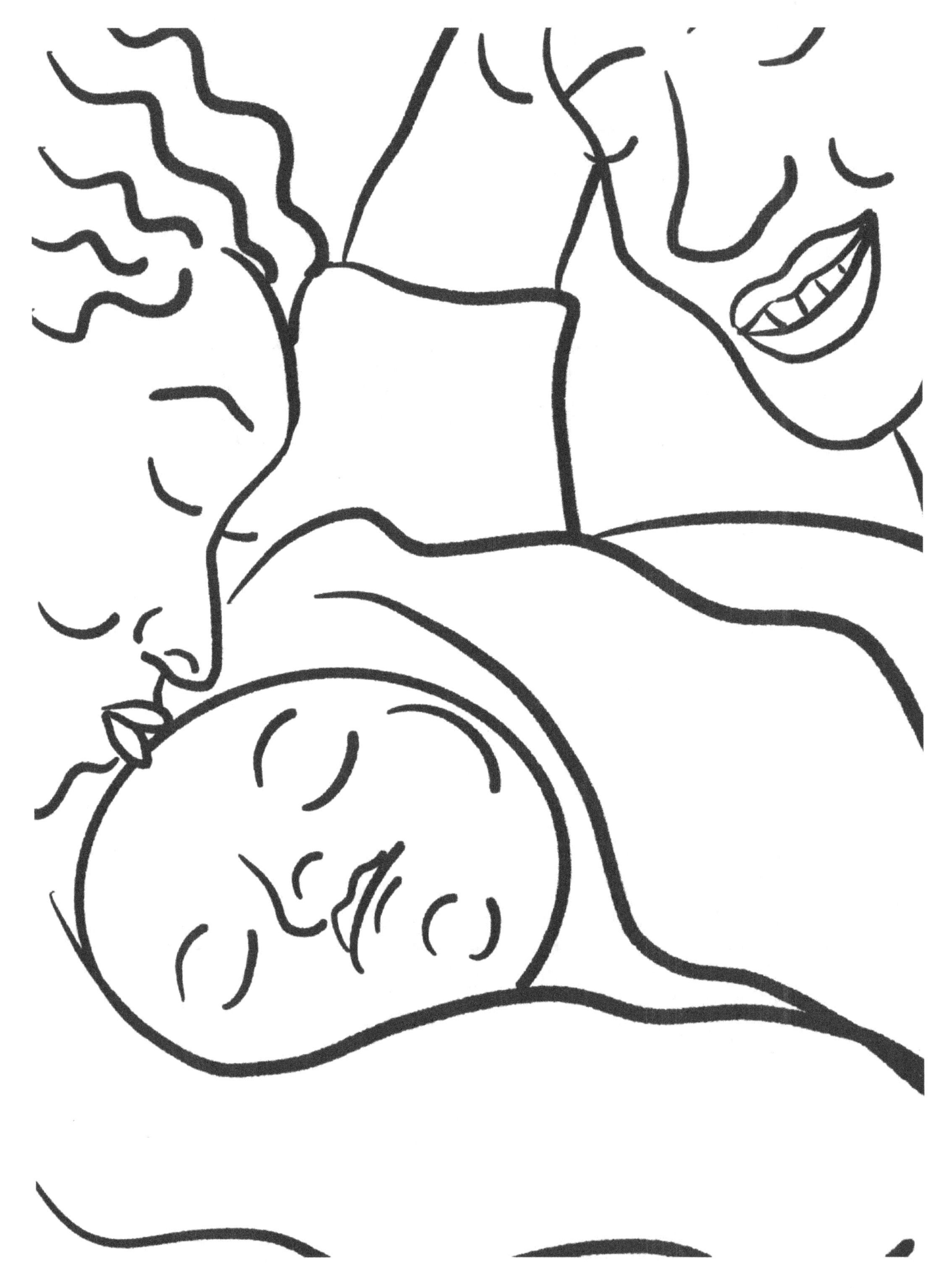

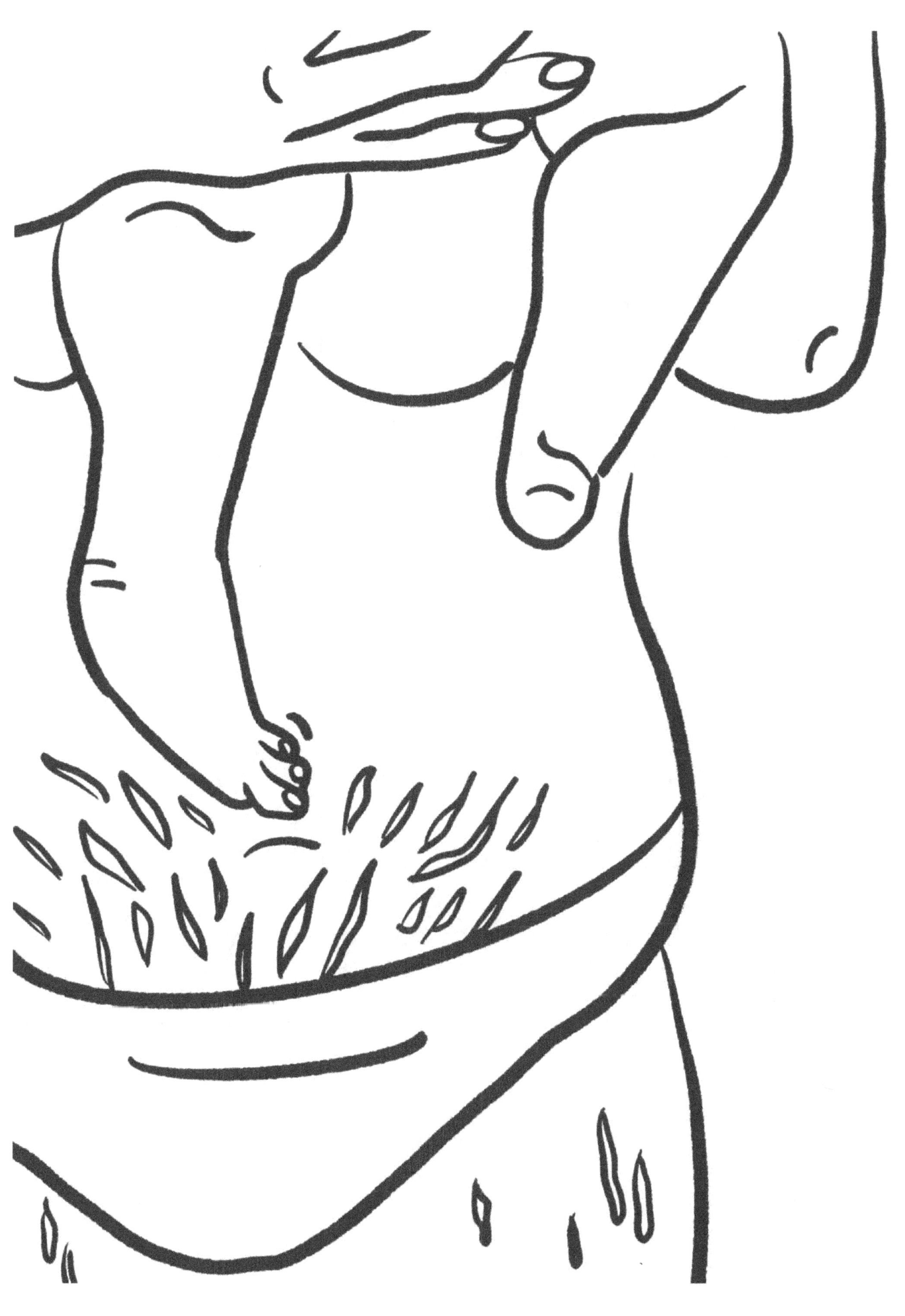

I CHOOSE TO LEARN TO LOVE AND THANK MY NEW BODY.

MY BIRTH EXPERIENCE IS BEAUTIFUL. NO MATTER HOW IT HAPPENS.